The Effective Charge Nurse Handbook

The Pocket Companion for Charge Nurse Leaders

Diana Swihart, PhD, DMin, MSN, APN CS, FAAN

Kelly J. Gantt, RN, MBA/HCM, BSN, VHA-CM

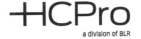

HCPro

a division of BLR

Diana Swihart, Author
Kelly J. Gantt, Author
Michelle Clarke, Editor
Erin Callahan, Vice President, Product Development & Content Strategy
Elizabeth Petersen, Executive Vice President, Healthcare
Matt Sharpe, Production Supervisor
Vincent Skyers, Design Services Director
Vicki McMahan, Sr. Graphic Designer
Jason Gregory, Layout/Graphic Design
Kelly Church, Cover Designer

Arrangements can be made for quantity discounts. For more information, contact:
HCPro
100 Winners Circle Suite 300
Brentwood, TN 37027
Telephone: 800-650-6787 or 781-639-1872
Fax: 800-785-9212
Email: *customerservice@hcpro.com*

Visit HCPro online at *www.hcpro.com* and *www.hcmarketplace.com*

Contents

About the Authors

Diana Swihart, PhD, DMin, MSN, APN CS, BC-RN, FAAN

Diana Swihart, PhD, DMin, MSN, APN CS, BC-RN, FAAN, is a consulting partner with the Forum for Shared Governance and the CEO and Managing Partner for the American Academy for Preceptor Advancement. She enjoys many roles in her professional career and practices in diverse clinical and nonclinical settings. An author, speaker, researcher, educator, and consultant, she has published and spoken nationally and internationally on a number of topics related to servant leadership, preceptors, shared governance, competency assessment, professional development, Magnet Recognition Program®, research, and evidence-based practice. In 2008, her publication *Nurse Preceptor Program Builder: Tools for a Successful Preceptor Program* (2nd ed.) was selected as a foundational resource for the national VHA RN Residency Program, now called the VHA RN Transition to Practice Program.

Dr. Swihart has served on the editorial advisory board for the *Journal of Nursing Regulation* and as an ANCC Magnet Recognition Program® appraiser, an ANCC Accreditation appraiser, the treasurer for the Association for Nursing Professional Development (prior to its name change), and adjunct faculty at South University and Trinity Theological Seminary and College of the Bible distance learning program. In 2015, Dr. Swihart was inducted as a Fellow into the American Academy of Nursing for her work in developing preceptor specialty practice and certification.

Kelly J. Gantt, MBA/HCM, BSN, VHA-CM

Kelly J. Gantt, MBA/HCM, BSN, VHA-CM, currently works as a Clinical Improvement Consultant and an academic facilitator for undergraduates and graduates focusing on Legal Issues in Health Care: Regulation and Compliance and Health Law and Ethics. She has a diverse experience in nursing, leadership, management, educator, and clinical roles within the healthcare industry (private, state, and federal entities). Gantt is innovative and instrumental in leading transformative initiatives that improve patient care and services.

With more than 18 years of proven versatility and adaptability, Gantt is adept in empowering and motivating others to be successful in performing above and beyond status quo and has a strong drive for excellence, continual learning, and new skill attainment. She is proficient in incorporating evidence-based practice into work performance and collaborating with other leaders. She provides education, training, facilitation, change management, quality improvement, performance improvement, patient safety, and project management. Skilled at managing operational and cultural complexity, she solves a broad range of problems effectively and generates ideas for process and systems improvement. Gantt is also a proud member of the Chi Eta Phi Sorority Inc., an international association for professional registered nurses.

Introduction

Leadership should be born out of the understanding of the needs of those who will be affected by it.

—Marion Anderson, Contralto Vocalist

About This Book

As a charge nurse, you lead in quality and patient safety, and you help manage costs of care in clinical microsystems within your organization. You navigate the intersections between staff, patients, families, and interdisciplinary care teams. As a registered nurse educated in the science of nursing and in the art of caring and administration, you must meet specified standards of education and clinical competence, and you must manage the operations of patient care units or areas during your assigned shifts. As a frontline leader, you support, mentor, guide, and evaluate patient care team members in providing safe, effective, efficient care.

In this role, you assume leadership of clinical operations and management of staff performance, work systems, and processes at the unit level to ensure safe, quality patient care is provided. Although you have limited formal leadership power, your impact on patient care and organizational outcomes is significant. Nurse managers depend on you to assume ever-expanding responsibilities for quality outcomes to meet multiple unit and organizational performance measures (Sherman, Schwarzkopf, & Kiger, 2011).

Although there is no one "right" development process approach for preparing charge nurses to be frontline leaders, this book aims to provide the following:

- The basic principles and ethics of frontline leadership
- The roles, responsibilities, and accountabilities of charge nurse leaders
- Tools to develop charge nurse leaders so they function effectively interprofessionally in diverse and demanding practice environments

How to Use This Book

This handbook will support your growth as a charge nurse in developing your confidence and skills in frontline leadership. It explores some basic skills and strategies.

In **Chapter 1: Preparing Charge Nurses to Lead**, we will look at the roles, responsibilities, and accountabilities for charge nurse leaders and compare management and leadership approaches; review the qualities and challenges inherent in the role; provide a sample job description; consider the principles of ethics in frontline leadership; and touch on the standards, requirements, and regulations that are part of a healthy workplace.

In **Chapter 2: Coordination and Delivery of Patient Care**, we discuss the patient flow process; managing patient safety; staffing and scheduling considerations; delegation and levels of authority, working with contract staff, agency staff, and unlicensed personnel; and managing documentation and patient care data, remembering to protect the information included even in end-of-shift reports.

In **Chapter 3: Managing Staff Performance**, we will explore ways to manage time and interruptions, facilitate change, communicate accurately and effectively, develop talent, problem solve using critical and creative thinking skills, and manage conflict while setting boundaries around incivility, bullying, and positional violence for a safe, productive workplace.

In **Chapter 4: Quality, Data, and Continual Improvement**, the world of quality improvement unfolds in your role in quality and continual improvement. It includes a few tools you can use for collecting, analyzing, displaying, and applying data to practice, and it outlines possibilities in partnering with Clinical Nurse Leaders to create a unit culture of safety, quality, and practice excellence.

In **Chapter 5: Performance Evaluations**, there are some tools and tips to help guide you and your team members in providing and receiving feedback, participating in performance evaluations, and successfully taking charge of your unit operations and coordination of patient care.

Finally, in **Chapter 6: Charge Nurse Leaders Caring for Self and Others**, we focus on the importance of caring for self in order to be able to continue caring for others, developing resiliency and managing stress, and engaging in intentional self-care.

We know how difficult, demanding, confusing, rewarding, and exhilarating the role of frontline leader can be. As a charge nurse leader, you wear many hats when managing your unit operations and coordinating patient care throughout your assigned shifts. You are the liaison between your nurse manager and team members; coordinator of team-based care; resource person for patients, families, and staff; and often the calm in the storms of conflict, creating a safe and healthy environment for caring. Use this handbook to encourage you and help you grow as a leader. It does not have all the answers, but hopefully, it will help you find the right questions.

1
Preparing Charge Nurses to Lead

Things are as they should be at this moment. When you accept
that, you become responsible for everything you have and are. You
then hold the power to change your future!
                                                                    —*Edward Lewellen*

Roles, Responsibilities, and Accountabilities for Charge Nurse Leaders

As a charge nurse leader, you wear many hats when managing your unit during your assigned shifts. Some assignments are permanent, and others only temporary, yet your responsibilities and accountabilities for the operations and patient outcomes during these times of service remain constant. Depending on your nurse manager, you often function as an adjunct to him or her with limited allocated authority.

Assessment exercise: This exercise will help you assess your current abilities and identify areas where you can learn and grow. Briefly describe the leadership skills you already have that enable you to meet assigned roles and responsibilities, such as the following. Place a check in the boxes of those you need to prepare you to lead in your practice setting:

- ❑ Transformational leadership
- ❑ Communication
- ❑ Teamwork
- ❑ Interprofessional collaborative practice (e.g., rounding, team-based care)
- ❑ Critical and creative systems thinking (e.g., coordination of care delivery systems)
- ❑ Accurate clinical judgment and decision-making
- ❑ Delegation
- ❑ Orientation, education, and competencies assessments
- ❑ Coach, preceptor, and mentor
- ❑ Clinician and nurse consultant for interprofessional partners and staff (i.e., stakeholder relationship building)
- ❑ Problem analysis and solution
- ❑ Time management
- ❑ Resource management (i.e., scheduling, staffing, material, and fiscal resources)
- ❑ Conflict management
- ❑ Advocacy and protection (i.e., navigating organizational and unit-level formal and informal rules)
- ❑ Stress management
- ❑ Planning and execution (e.g., regulatory requirements, care assignments, admissions and discharges, student activities)
- ❑ Managing staff performance (e.g., performance appraisals, peer reviews)
- ❑ Continual quality and performance improvement
- ❑ Motivation and team building
- ❑ Succession planning

Now that you have a better idea of your own strengths and needs for developing your charge nurse leader skills, what kind of manager or leader are you? What kind do you want to be?

Comparing Management and Leadership Approaches

Leaders are people who do the right thing; managers are people who do things right. Both roles are crucial, and they differ profoundly.
—*Warren Bennis, Leadership Author*

Charge nurse leaders both manage and lead, depending on the need or situation. However, there are differences in the roles and functions of management and leadership. Let's take a brief look at some of the elements of traditional management and collaborative leadership approaches:

- *Traditional management approach*: This is a more transactional, directive, or parental management style:
  - Focuses on managing tasks and is compliance driven.
  - Relies on patriarchal and autocratic traditions; "power over" attitudes and practices

- *Collaborative leadership approach*: Transformational leadership is genuine, collaborative, and process-driven:
  - Position used to remain involved clinically and administratively while influencing and shaping patient outcomes
  - Provides support, guidance, coaching and mentoring, safety, feedback, and work-specific performance assessments to staff and healthcare team members around patient-centered care

Today's workforce responds less well to traditional approaches by charge nurse leaders and calls for transformational leaders at every level of nursing service across the organization. Leadership is integrated into team-based care, with charge nurse leaders facilitating the operations of their assigned units throughout their shifts. Team-based care is essentially a relational, communal process.

As you gain increasing insight into your role delineation, responsibilities, accountabilities, and ability to influence performance, it is essential to develop your leadership skills as quickly as possible. Porter-O'Grady (2003) defined leadership as a multifaceted process of identifying goals and targets, motivating others to act, and providing support and motivation to achieve mutually negotiated goals. What qualities do you need for the charge nurse leader role? What challenges might you expect to encounter along the way?

Charge Nurse Leader Qualities and Challenges

Sherman, Schwarzkopf, and Kiger (2011; 2013) identified five themes with concomitant qualities for charge nurse leaders:

1. Manage communication: Actively listen, keep others updated and current, and remain sensitive to diverse styles of communication and cultural differences in meanings and language

2. Act as a team coach: Remain clinically competent, act as a resource person and educator, and collaborate and delegate appropriately and fairly

3. Be seen as approachable: Be empathetic and nonjudgmental, give and receive feedback accurately and with compassion, and remain transparent and accessible

4. Work like an air traffic controller: Organize, prioritize, and

delegate effectively and efficiently, manage unit and service chaos, and reduce stress levels among team members

5. Be professional at all times: Assume accountability for actions, be confident and diplomatic with interprofessional and interdisciplinary team members, and maintain a leadership presence with respect and advocacy

At the same time, recognize that you can and will confront a multitude of challenges in your frontline leadership role. Significant challenges include but are not limited to the following:

- Conflict and workplace violence
- Patient and family satisfaction
- A safe patient care environment
- Delegation
- Communication
- Rapidly changing policies, procedures, and regulations
- Increasingly complex regulatory requirements
- Supervision and decision-making
- Coaching, preceptoring (especially new staff), feedback, and evaluations
- Patient care assignments and patient transfers

Additionally, you need lifelong learning to advance your communication, collaboration, and collegiality skills to meet the present and future challenges of increasingly complex healthcare and work environments. First, you have to know what the job requires.

Charge Nurse Leader Job Description

Not every nurse can be a frontline leader. Some facilities provide job descriptions for the charge nurse leader role (see Figure 1.1), which provide a standardized foundation for consistent expectations, qualifications and competencies, and evaluations of performance.

Job descriptions or functional statements clarify the qualities you need to be successful, but they do not address the unique challenges of unit leadership. To discover those, you will collaborate with your nurse manager to do the following:

- Set goals and targets for your leadership and team activities,
- Identify the levels of authority and accountability given to you for interacting with staff and team members
- Determine how and when to communicate problems, reports and outcomes.

Successful operations of the shift and unit staff, team morale and motivation, management of difficult or challenging situations, and maintenance of open lines of communication depend on your professional qualities and abilities to meet leadership challenges in managing the team and operations of your unit or practice setting during your assigned shifts.

Figure 1.1 Charge nurse leader job description (sample)

Charge nurse leader job description	
Job title	Charge nurse leader
Job category	Nursing services
Job code	(Job code #)
Location	(Hospital location)
Department	(Department location)
Position type	Full-time weekdays; (3) 12-hour shifts

Fig 1.1 Charge nurse leader job description (sample) (cont.)

Level	RN Level III

Position summary

The charge nurse leader is responsible for the assessment, coordination, implementation, and evaluation of the delivery of safe and effective patient-centered care during her or his assigned shift. The charge nurse leader will facilitate, preceptor, and mentor staff and team members to grow professionally and advance their knowledge and skills. S/he will continuously assess unit needs to ensure adequate resources for current and upcoming shifts by collaborating with other departments, clinical and nonclinical, to coordinate timely admissions, transfers, and discharges of patients. The charge nurse leaders will demonstrate professionalism at all times, meet regulatory and policy requirements, engage standards of practice, and hold team members accountable for safe, competent practice, quality care, and continual improvement.

Qualifications summary

- ❑ Current nursing license
- ❑ Current Basic Life Support (BLS) certificate
- ❑ Current Advanced Cardiac Life Support (ACLS) certificate (if appropriate)
- ❑ Minimum baccalaureate degree in nursing
- ❑ Two years' work experience in assigned area of practice or patient population

Competency summary

- ❑ Demonstrates an understanding of regulatory requirements and professional practice guidelines
- ❑ Presents a working knowledge of organizational policies and procedures
- ❑ Shows competence in the performance of unit-specific skills to be a resource and mentor for team members
- ❑ Demonstrates knowledge and skills in the following:

  - • Communication
  - • Conflict management
  - • Time management
  - • Leadership
  - • Stress management
  - • Computer technology, i.e., Outlook, Microsoft Word, Excel, Team building and Computerized Patient Records Systems

Fig 1.1 Charge nurse leader job description (sample) (cont.)

Duties and responsibilities

- ❑ Set the tone for a productive, professional work environment
- ❑ Remain knowledgeable of all technical duties and responsibilities for area of expertise
- ❑ Participate in interdepartmental and hospital performance improvement activities
- ❑ Proactively round with team members in the unit and identify opportunities for improvement
- ❑ Collaborate with other departments in a professional manner to deliver safe, quality patient-centered care
- ❑ Provide a safe, clean, and secure work and practice environment
- ❑ Monitor utilization of equipment and supplies and ensure safety and availability; follow hospital policy
- ❑ Assist in evaluating staff and ensure that mandatory education is complete
- ❑ Assign and delegate patient care tasks as appropriate, considering staff members, level of nursing experience, competency, and knowledge
- ❑ Collaborate with the clinical educator planning and evaluating nursing staff
- ❑ Address performance issues appropriately while treating employees consistently, fairly, and respectfully
- ❑ Promote, facilitate, and provide education about new practice changes, regulatory requirements, and organizational policies to team members on the unit
- ❑ Assume role of patient care manager in his or her absence
- ❑ Actively participate on unit-based shared governance councils
- ❑ Report to a member of the leadership team in a timely manner all significant events such as near misses, never and adverse events, complaints, and any situation affecting safe delivery of patient-centered care
- ❑ Ensure that handover communication occurs any time there is a change in caregivers on the unit throughout the shift and during change of shift
- ❑ Remain fiscally responsible at all times; ensure appropriate staffing levels for unit and departmental needs, monitor supplies, and manage equipment

Fig 1.1 Charge nurse leader job description (sample) (cont.)

- ❑ Demonstrate effective communication, conflict management, people management, and team-building activities
- ❑ Participate in updating and upholding standards of practice; role model to others by maintaining the ethical standards of behavior
- ❑ Adhere to professional guidelines for practice such as State Board of Nursing and the American Nurses Association professional standards of care
- ❑ Assist in monitoring staff performance, behavior, and competency for performance reviews

Additional requirements

- ❑ Attends at least 70% of monthly staff meetings
- ❑ Participates in at least two process improvement projects annually
- ❑ Preceptors other charge nurse leaders to the position as needed
- ❑ Obtains a national certification in the area of specialty, if available, within the first year of the position
- ❑ Attends ongoing leadership training courses offered by the facility as required for the position

Reporting structure

- • Reports to the nurse manager or unit supervisor

Signatures/Initials

Source: Adapted from *Charge Nurse Leader Program Builder, 2nd Edition* © 2015 HCPro.

Ethics for Charge Nurses in Frontline Leadership

Like your practice, your frontline leadership requires you adhere to ethical principles (ANA, 2015). There is value added when you practice within your professional code of ethics and abide by policies, facility ethics guidelines, and legal standards, such as employee confidentiality. You often serve as advocate, negotiator, protector, preceptor, and counselor to team members, patients, and families. Additionally, you help new staff members settle into their new roles and positions and may preceptor or mentor students completing clinical assignments on your unit.

A *code of ethics* is a set of principles of conduct within an organization that guides decision-making and behavior (Makaroff, Storch, Pauly, & Newton, 2014). Applying ethical, legal, and policy rules is essential to safe, effective nursing practice and leadership. Most ethics codes specify members conduct themselves honestly, fairly, competently, and justly.

Ethics exercise: This exercise will help you consider some potential ethical questions and principles you may encounter as a frontline leader and ways to anticipate them with proactive problem solving (Gantt, 2014):

- Read your specialty practice or profession's code of ethics: What issues are discussed? What were the outcomes? What might be done differently?

- Draw on personal, practical, lived experiences: What about a situation or question was troubling? Review the Choice and Awareness Model (Figure 1.2) and consider how it might apply to the ethics of the discussion or situation. This model offers one approach for ethical decision-making and working through ethical dilemmas. What other models have you used?

- Look through books and journals on ethics that include situations testing personal or professional values, beliefs, or morals in how to perform work or interact with co-workers, colleagues, or customers/clients/patients. How do these examples fit situations you encountered during a preceptorship or mentorship? How will your decisions be affected by the ethical choices made by those in the books or journals?

We are all guided by basic ethical principles (see Figure 1.3). These principles and how they are interpreted and folded into practice are an important part of any code of conduct you embrace as a frontline leader (ANA, 2015).

Figure 1.2 Ethical choice and awareness model

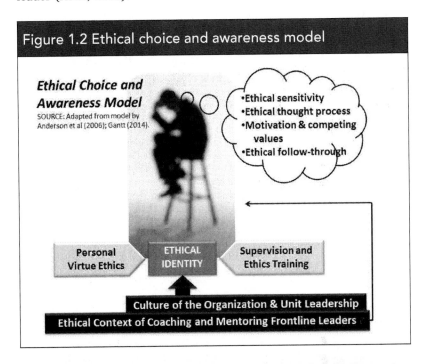

Figure 1.3 Ethical principles for charge nurse leaders

Ethical principles		
Focus	Definition	Examples for charge nurse leaders
Autonomy	Personal freedom, right of self-determination	Provide only the guidance required to be successful and allow for exploration, trial and error, and the opportunity to fail forward as they develop their own competencies in knowledge and skills

Fig. 1.3 Ethical principles for charge nurse leaders (cont.)

Beneficence	Duty to have the best interests of the recipient or participant as the goal of any actions or decisions	Assist them in understanding the legal and ethical standards that apply to their leadership duties to ensure safe, competent, and beneficial work-related activities
Non-maleficence	Duty to prevent intentional harm from occurring; sometimes combined with beneficence and presented as a single ethical principle and based on the Hippocratic maxim, "First do no harm"	Test decisions and actions by asking, "Could my decision or actions cause harm in any way?"
Veracity	Truth-telling	Engage in honest, bi-directional feedback and encouragement; support concerns and invite questions; explore false conduct or misrepresentations, behaviors, and comments immediately to correct any deviations from truth
Justice	Fairness, treating all equally	All actions and decisions are just and guided by truth, reason, equity, and fairness for all participants (i.e., staff, other team members, managers, educators, students, families, patients, etc.)

Fig. 1.3 Ethical principles for charge nurse leaders (cont.)		
Paternalism	Telling others what is best, often without considering their input; the practice of treating or governing people in a fatherly (paternal) manner; a form of control versus influence over behaviors and actions	Charge nurse leaders who want to help, advise, or protect may neglect individual choice and personal responsibility, causing staff, team members, or patients, for example, to become disengaged in the process; often seen in transactional leadership
Fidelity	Duty to keep one's promises and commitments	Provide factual accuracy in reporting information and keep promises, e.g., keep appointments with staff and other team members, follow up with agreed-upon tasks, and provide timely feedback
Respect for others	Duty to treat all with thoughtfulness, with consideration, and without prejudice	Determine which rules, obligations, and values should direct choices; recognize the abilities of others, e.g., when respecting another's judgment in a given situation

Navigating Regulatory Standards, Requirements, and Regulations

> *It is essential to know which driving factors are coming from external standards and which are coming from internal organizational policies.*
>
> —*Donna Wright*

All organizations and professions adhere to regulatory standards of practice, and the healthcare industry is no exception. Every healthcare organization is guided by regulatory standards, standards of practice, and codes of ethics. They must uphold state, governmental, and other regulatory agency guidelines. Regulatory agencies guide practice and safety while attempting to mitigate risks to patients and providers. As a charge nurse leader, you will frequently be called upon to educate staff and team members on standards of practice and regulatory guidelines for your unit and the care you manage.

The U.S. Patient Protection and Affordable Care Act (ACA) is changing the landscape of healthcare. As a systems thinker, you must consider the current and future impact of ACA on hospital-based healthcare. Sherman (2012) identified five ways that the ACA could change nursing:

1. Increased nursing workforce needs

2. An expansion of nursing roles outside of acute care

3. A need for more Nurse Practitioners

4. Increased accountability for healthcare quality and value

5. Opportunities for development of innovative nursing care delivery models

The ANA (2012) analyzed the ACA legislation and determined it will change nursing. They urged nurse leaders to be proactive in planning for the changes. You are in a key position to partner with your nurse manager and senior nurse leaders to facilitate these changes proactively.

As a frontline leader within a healthcare organization, you have a professional responsibility to practice and role model the behaviors that support a healthy unit or work area in delivering reliable and safe high-quality patient care. Participate in your professional organizations, review professional journals and monitor trends and issues in healthcare to forecast changes, share research and evidence-based practice, and explore innovative strategies and solutions related to nursing regulation and practice. When rounding and during team meetings (Swihart & Gantt, 2015), discuss the many operational processes, standards, regulations, and policies that affect patient-centered care, such as the following:

- Patient-centered care
- Patient satisfaction
- Service recovery
- Regulating ethics
- State and regulatory standards
- Scope and standards of nursing practice
- The Joint Commission

Healthy workplaces do not just happen. It is important for you to feel safe in your charge nurse leader role, to have resources and organizational support in managing unit or work area operations, to feel supported, and to know your concerns will be addressed. Partner with your nurse manager to facilitate team building and open communication among staff and team members and address operational situations, as in the following example:

Nurse/patient ratios. Comparable and sufficient nurse/patient ratios are a national issue in nursing practice. Charge nurse leaders generally make and manage patient assignment. Ensuring that an assignment is appropriate requires teamwork, open communication, and a safe environment where nurses are able to express their concerns about workload balance, consistency of care assignments, and staff and patent safety. If a nurse does not feel that an assignment is safe, for example, you as the charge nurse leader are expected to actively listen to the concerns being expressed and either make necessary changes or consult with your nurse manager or hospital supervisor for guidance. The process and outcomes used to mitigate the stated concern of the nurse(s) must then be clearly documented according to the organization's policy.

Most organizations adhere to the regulatory requirements of agencies such as The Joint Commission, state Boards of Nursing, Centers for Medicare & Medicaid Services, professional standards of practice and care, codes of ethical conduct, and administrative and clinical facility policies and procedures, such as handover communication processes. Reviewing and adhering to them is truly like navigating the whitewaters of legislation, regulation, accreditation, standards, rules and laws, and policies: You cannot do it alone. It is important to learn about those used in your organization, on your unit, and by your team members. Explore them with your nurse manager, educators, preceptors, and mentors—they are the ones who will prepare you to know when to manage and how to truly lead.

2

Coordination and Delivery of Patient Care

We often think of nursing as giving meds on time, checking an X-ray to see if the doctor needs to be called, or taking an admission at 2:00 a.m. with a smile on our faces. Too often, we forget all the other things that make our job what it truly is: caring and having a desire to make a difference.

—*Erin Pettengill*

Many nurses go to work every day, accept their assignments, care for their patients, document care and medications in the medical record, report changes, and update the charge nurse leader and oncoming nurses for the next shift. More is expected of the charge nurse leader. You coordinate and deliver effective patient-centered care as part of the operations of your unit and team. You assess and make schedules and assignments; anticipate and mitigate unit risks and conflict; manage patient flow, supplies, and resources; and ensure patient satisfaction and safety. To better understand these roles and responsibilities, let's start by discussing the patient flow process.

Patient Flow Process

Few hospital areas are designed to achieve optimal flow of patients. Major bottlenecks include the emergency department, intensive care units, and operating rooms and their related pre- and post-care areas. You cannot unclog these bottlenecks in isolation. You can help improve flow by reducing the process variation that impacts it by facilitating the smooth movement of patients through acute care settings. Although some variability is normal, other variances are not and can be eliminated. The Institute for Healthcare Improvement (IHI, 2003) recommended that frontline leadership (yes, that's you) do the following:

- Evaluate flow and move patients through the system in a timely and efficient manner

- Measure and evaluate variability from all sources, such as waiting times for tests and procedures, medication delivery times, physician rounds, ebb and flow of patient admissions, transfers, discharges throughout the day, and professional variability among team members (e.g., competencies and skill levels among staff and providers; staffing levels and ratios)

- Consider process changes that could result from collaborative relationships with other services and departments (e.g., pharmacy, social services, dietetics, radiology, therapy departments; consistent timing of scheduled procedures for patients and when physicians make rounds on the unit)

- Provide a process for giving advance notice and scheduling when patients will be transferred from the unit or discharged; manage the transfer or discharge accordingly

Patient flow engages the whole system of care, not just nursing units or work areas. Organizations maintain patient flow mapping plans, which describe the types of services offered by nursing and how the services interact with other service lines. This flow map visualizes the whole process a patient will experience from the time of admission to the time of discharge.

When care is provided is as important as what care is provided. Facilitate discussions with staff and other team members to reduce variabilities and improve patient flow as much as possible within the unit. Plan ahead. Learn to identify patterns that disrupt patient flow. Seek solutions proactively through interprofessional and interdisciplinary collaborations with other departments. Unexpected bottlenecks and variances in patient flow impact patient safety.

Managing Patient Safety

Patient safety is woven into every aspect of unit operations and coordination and delivery of patient care. The charge nurse leader must be transparent about unit performance measures, process improvements, data management, and reporting. Some of your key activities influence patient safety, such as emergency management and emergency documentation, errors and near misses, and data collection. Two nursing interventions—patient rounding and end-of-shift reporting—enhance patient safety.

Both structured and "as needed" rounding ensure timely responses and promote patient satisfaction and safety. Rounding serves as a means to communicate with patients and families, to visually assess the environment to determine if it is safe, and often sets the stage for what goals need to be achieved during the shift. End-of-shift reporting by staff to charge nurse leaders is a common practice for summarizing patient care issues that may impact the unit and need to be communicated to the oncoming charge nurse leader. End-of-shift report is often a table-top activity away from patients and families. Therefore, you may only hear rather than experience what the staff is reporting. If you do not already have a standard form, the sample charge nurse leader shift report form (see figure 2.1) offers one way to organize the information collected during the end-of-shift report. Combining these two interventions has proven to be a useful way to enhance patient safety, interprofessional communication, and teamwork, while keeping you accessible to staff and patients.

Figure 2.1 Charge nurse leader shift report (sample)

Unit:	Shift:					
Date:						
Subject	**Report**					
Staffing	RN	LPN/LVN	UAP	CNL	APN	Others
Day shift						
Evening shift						
Night shift						
Number of patients						
Patient acuity levels						
Resuscitation status						
Pre- and post-op patients						
Admissions						
Transfers						

Figure 2.1 Charge nurse leader shift report (sample) (cont.)	
Discharges	
Special procedures and treatments	
Critical tests and results	
High-risk concerns for monitoring or follow-up	
Staff concerns	
Notes	

Source: Adapted from *Charge Nurse Leader Program Builder, 2nd Edition* © 2015 HCPro.

Staffing and Scheduling

Staffing and scheduling are variables to patient flow. If there is not enough staff to meet patient care demand, the safe and timely delivery of patient care is adversely affected. These important responsibilities have multiple components: patient classification systems, staffing mix, distribution of staff, flexibility, and other support staff. Work closely with your nurse manager or other nurse leaders to learn the policies and guidelines for managing staffing and schedules on your unit until you are comfortable with the process. Let's briefly look at what is involved:

- **Patient classification systems (PCS), or patient acuity systems,** are used to forecast unit staffing needs and to determine workload requirements. Acuity levels identify how much nursing assistance patients; the more nursing assistance they need, the higher the acuity.
- **Staffing mix and distribution of staffing** are determined by current patient needs each shift. **The ANA *Principles for Nurse Staffing* (2012)** is an excellent resource for learning more about your professional accountability and responsibility in staffing.

Patient acuity systems, staffing levels and mixes, and scheduling are about managing operations effectively, coordinating activities and services, and ensuring the delivery of safe and timely patient-centered care.

Delegation and Levels of Authority

As a frontline leader, you participate in shared decision-making with your nurse manager, team members, and patients. To be successful in your charge nurse leader role, you need the autonomy and authority to make and determine the appropriateness of your own decisions and delegated tasks and assignments. You will be most successful in confidently making decisions when your responsibility, authority, and accountability (R + A + A) are clearly delineated and assigned (Wright, 2002). But what exactly do those look like?

Responsibility is the clear and specific allocation of duties to achieve desired results. Assignment of responsibility is a two-way process: It is visibly given and visibly accepted. Acceptance is the essence of responsibility. However, individuals cannot accept responsibility without a level of authority.

Authority is the right to act and make decisions in the areas where one is given and accepts responsibility. When people are asked to share in the work, they must know their level of authority for carrying out that work. "Levels of authority" describe the right to act in areas given and to accept authority based on the situation; they must be given to those who are asked to take on responsibility. There are four levels of authority:

1. *Data gathering*: "Get information, bring it back to me, and I will decide what to do with it."

2. *Data gathering + recommendations*: "Get the information (collect the data), look at the situation and make some recommendations, and I will pick from one of those recommendations what we will do next. I still decide."

3. *Data gathering + recommendations [pause] + act*: "Get the information (collect the data), look at the situation and make some recommendations, and pick one that you will do. But before you carry it out, I want you to stop (pause) and check with me before you do it." The pause is not necessarily for approval. It is more of a double check, to make sure that everything was considered before proceeding.

4. *Act and inform or update*: "Do what needs to be done, and tell me what happened or update me later." There is no pause before the action.

Accountability begins when you review and reflect upon your own actions and decisions, and it culminates with a personal assessment that helps determine the best actions to take in the future. *Accountability cannot be delegated.*

Delegation is the transfer of responsibility for the performance of a specific task. In every delegation decision, you must use accurate nursing judgement and provide appropriate supervision when needed. Regardless of who delegated a nursing task, any team member who observes another person performing a patient care task incorrectly must withdraw the delegation and report any actions taken in accordance with policy, procedure, standard, or law. As the charge nurse leader, you provide delegatees with initial and ongoing direction, guidance, observation, and evaluation of the performance of the delegated task.

Charge nurse leaders are accountable, answerable, and liable for their own actions, for completing assigned tasks, and acts of delegation to team members. To learn how to delegate effectively and accurately, use a delegation tool and process worksheet (see Figure 2.2). You may also delegate tasks to contract staff, agency nurses, or unlicensed assistive personnel. However, to do so effectively, ensure that you know something about these other team members and what can or cannot be delegated to them.

Figure 2.2 Sample charge nurse leader delegation tool

Charge nurse leader delegation tool	
Name:	**Date:**
Situation to be delegated	
Level of authority delegated	
Objective(s) What do you want the team member to do?	

Figure 2.2 Sample charge nurse leader shift report form (cont.)

Critical steps to be used What steps are necessary to complete the task or assignment? When?	
Background information Facts known Information needed Concerns Possible causes or reason(s) for the situation Previous discussions Consequences if the situation continues Other	
Alternatives Possible actions Possible solutions Resources available Constraints Other	

Summary notes

Specific actions	Person responsible	By when

Follow-up Date, time, place Other	

Figure 2.2 Sample charge nurse leader delegation tool (cont.)

Review

To what extent did you meet your objectives?

What did you handle most effectively?

What could you have used more effectively?

What will you do differently next time?

Delegation process worksheet

Task or assignment	Possible strategies
1. Describe the task or assignment Be specific Focus on facts, actions, issues Avoid interfering with team member	
2. Ask for obstacles for completing the task or assignment Use open-ended questions Listen attentively	
3. Respond as needed Stress that the task/assignment must be completed Address mutual benefits Listen and respond with empathy	
4. Discuss possible solutions Use person's ideas, when appropriate Listen and respond with empathy	
5. Agree on specific action and follow-up State who, what, when Check for understanding Listen and respond with empathy	

Figure 2.2 Sample charge nurse leader delegation tool (cont.)	
6. Express appreciation for the person's willingness to handle the situation Be sincere End on a positive note Maintain or enhance self-esteem	

Working with Contract Staff, Agency Staff, and Unlicensed Personnel

When delegating tasks and making assignments, consider team members who are contract or agency staff and unlicensed assistive personnel. Make sure that you have a description of these roles and responsibilities and that you know what your accountabilities are relative to these caregivers' delivery of services. When making assignments, some helpful documents to have include the following:

- A copy of their completed partial or full hospital orientation to the organization and facility policies
- Their service-specific orientation to the unit
- Contract and agency staff records of training and competency from their employers listing their skills and abilities
- Facility or unit guidelines and a list of what contract and agency staff are eligible to work on your unit
- A list of agencies the organization uses and the qualified agency staff members who are able to work in the organization or department

Unlicensed assistive personnel usually refers to the students, patient care technicians or aides, or nursing assistants who work on units and help with basic patient care needs (e.g., baths, feedings, vital signs, bed changes, and so on). They provide care that does not require a licensed practical/vocational nurse or registered nurse's advanced skills and knowledge. They are often assigned to partner with licensed nurses in providing patient care.

Managing Documentation and Patient Care Data

As a charge nurse leader, your responsibilities include reports, patient care records, computerized medical records, and other forms of documentation that are part of managing unit operations and coordinating patient care. Organize your information so it remains confidential, accessible, and understandable by those receiving it. amiliarize yourself with the regulatory issues of handover communication, change-of-shift patient reports, and anecdotal information about staffing, number of patients, number of anticipated admissions, discharges and transfers, patient acuity levels, resuscitation status, special procedures and treatments, critical tests and results, and any high-risk concerns for monitoring or follow-up. In long-term care facilities, the plan of care is often discussed, such as discharge planning or treatment plans, and the disciplines that are involved.

The security of patient information is everyone's responsibility. Be very careful with your end-of-shift reports—they contain critical and often confidential patient care data that must be protected. Shred your notes before leaving the unit, or place them in a safe area until they are no longer needed. If there is any breach in confidentiality, assess the situation. Follow your facility policies and procedures, and contact the appropriate staff immediately.

3
Managing Staff Performance

All of us spend time doing ridiculous things that are a complete waste of time simply to avoid going out of our comfort zone.
—Dr. Stephen Covey

Managing Time and Interruptions

In his *Seven Habits of Highly Effective People* (2004), Stephen Covey presented a matrix with four quadrants that can help you learn how to manage your time and meetings more effectively. His schematic explains how to put first things first by identifying different levels of urgency and importance—even for activities that are unpleasant. All time can be divided into one of these four quadrants. The matrix in Figure 3.1 places typical leadership activities and responsibilities into each of the four quadrants. Categorizing work honestly helps you organize, prioritize, and delegate appropriately in your charge nurse leader role (Sherman, 2013).

Figure 3.1 Time prioritization matrix		
	Urgent	**Not Urgent**
Important	**I** • Crises • Pressing problems • Deadline driven projects, meetings, preparations	**II** • Preparations • Presentations • Values clarifications • Planning • Relationship building • True recreation • Empowerment
Not Important	**III** • Interruptions, some phone calls • Some mail, some reports, some meetings • Many proximate pressing matters • Many popular activities	**IV** • Trivia, busywork • Junk mail • Some phone calls • Time wasters • "Escape" activities

To lead people effectively and manage unit operations efficiently, the three most important time management skills are organization, prioritization, and delegation (Swihart & Figueroa, 2014):

- *Organization* is more than a list of tasks. It includes scheduling meetings, interruptions, rounding, and time with staff and other team members to give and receive feedback, concerns, and ideas for improving unit operations. Set aside time during the shift to update reports. Complete each task before beginning a new one.

- *Prioritization* is identifying urgent tasks, completing what *must* be completed during a shift, and determining what can be done later or may not be necessary. What do you need to focus on or prioritize to achieve unit and patient care outcomes for your shift? Use an end-of-shift report (see Figure 2.1) to assess the tasks and duties that can be responsibly and safely managed.

Charge Nurse Program Builder

- *Delegation* (see Chapter 2) is the transfer of responsibility for the performance of a specific task. Remember, accountability CANNOT be delegated.

Interruptions and distractions in clinical settings present unnecessary risks to staff and patients. Therefore, you must manage your time as efficiently as you manage your duties. This is especially true when you are facilitating change.

Facilitating Change

Every role creates change. You are an experienced clinician with varying levels of proficiency in leading unit operations and coordinating team-based patient-centered care. However, you may be unsure of your skills and abilities when stepping into a more administrative role as a charge nurse leader. In addition, even temporarily assuming the responsibility of managing the unit in a nurse manager's absence or under his or her leadership can be a jarring change in the status quo. Peers are no longer peers but team members and staff. You now have supervisory responsibilities, such as staffing and scheduling, making assignments, and managing patient flow.

Change is a dynamic process. It always causes some degree of conflict or resistance, but it also may stimulate positive behaviors and attitudes. *Change management* is a process for making changes in a deliberate, planned, systematic manner to adapt to new experiences, roles, duties, and accountabilities. When facilitating change on the unit, it is important to ease people through real and perceived concerns (Swihart & Figueroa, 2014):

- Prepare and plan the changes with the staff and team members

- Identify who will support and who will oppose the changes
- Define timelines and tradeoffs
- Use team meetings, in-services, and other formats for planning, implementing, and communicating the change with team members
- Communicate factually, comprehensively, and frequently
- Consider expectations, risks, and the potential of failure
- Remember, people react differently to change; basic needs influence reaction to change
- Manage changes realistically; deal with fears, expectations, and concerns honestly

Manage strategic change based on environmental scanning, forecasting, evolving regulations, mandates, and practice requirements. The key to successful change lies with those who see the need for change, make the needed changes (move), and follow through with the changes (finish). Black and Gregersen (2008) urge leaders to change the individual first (e.g., potential charge nurse leaders) and services, departments, and organizations will follow. You are in a key position to help your team members and patients see that change truly can be a good thing when done well. Let change begin with you.

Communicating Accurately and Effectively

When we listen with the intent to understand others, rather than with the intent to reply, we begin true communication and relationship building. Opportunities to then speak openly and to be understood [take] consideration; seeking to be understood takes courage. Effectiveness lies in balancing the two.

—*Stephen Covey*

Tanzi (2015) described *communication* as "a complex, intricately woven, dynamic, and fluid construct of verbal and nonverbal cues interpreted (and often misinterpreted) through multidimensional filters (e.g., culture, generations, gender, perception, education, and lived experiences)" (p. 144). The only absolute is that it is impossible NOT to communicate through gestures, emotion, behaviors (e.g., distancing), and touch.

The purpose of communication is to create shared understanding. Although interpersonal communication is often referred to as "one to one" communication, it actually encompasses the exchange of information between two or more persons. This is seen, for example, when communication occurs between two or more nurses assigned to a patient with multiple co-morbidities, and it may include other stakeholders (e.g., educators, staff, other team members, and interprofessional partners), as well.

Communication is transmitted in four primary forms: written, spoken (verbal), nonverbal, and visualizations. Rounding is an example of when all four forms may be used to report details of a patient's status, care delivery, and prognosis:

- *Written communication*: Reports, data sheets, charting (e.g., pharmacy and medical records), end-of-shift reports, interviews, surveys, academic papers, letters, books, magazines, internet, and other forms of media
- *Spoken or verbal communications*: Voice tone and pitch, language, face-to-face (FTF), telephones, radios, television, internet (e.g., computer programs, videos, and movies), and other forms of media
- *Nonverbal communication*: Gestures, body language, posture, personal space
- *Visualizations*: Graphs, charts, posters, maps, logos, pictures, and other venues for communicating information, messages, and branding

Barriers to accurate communication distort or corrupt intended messages. These include perception, message, emotion, language, culture, bias, age, pain, environmental distractions, assumptions, stress, fear, health, and self-talk (i.e., background noise). You need strong interpersonal skills to transcend the many filters that can sabotage your ability to communicate effectively—words and gestures can hurt or heal. Professional jargon creates barriers to collaborative interprofessional patient-centered care; wheras, tools such as SBAR (Situation-Background-Assessment-Recommendation), call-outs, check-backs, write-down read-back, and handovers enhance accurate communication in clinical practice.

Freeman Teague, Jr., assured us "Nothing is so simple that it cannot be misunderstood." Clarification and accuracy are vital to all forms of communication. Readily and consistently engage in honest, open discussions and teaching and learning moments. Clarifying responses such as "What I hear you saying is ..." or "If I understand you correctly ..." demonstrate genuineness and an attempt to accurately capture the intended message. Positive reinforcement statements might include such words as "I really liked the way you ..."; "next time you will be even better if you ..."; "tell me what you thought went well during that (assignment, procedure, assessment, activity)." Choose your messages and responses with careful intent, compassion, and discretion at all times to ensure clear, accurate, and consistent communication.

Developing Talent

A leader's lasting legacy will not be measured by the buildings we build, the institutions we establish, or what our team accomplished. Leaders are judged by how well the people they invest in carry on after they are gone.

—*John C. Maxwell*

Sherman (2013) asks, "Where have all the Nurse Leaders gone?" and more critically, perhaps, who will take their place. Hospitals, nurse leaders, and professional organizations are asking the same questions. Succession planning happens in many ways but often begins at points of service. Nurses coach, preceptor, and mentor students, peers, and colleagues with leadership potential and interest. For example, your nurse manager may have actively sought out employees with the skill and motivation to become charge nurse leaders and found you. Although not all nurse leaders do this or engage in succession planning and talent development, great leaders do. They honor and nurture the goals and aspirations of their employees, recognizing the potential greatness in every nurse.

Talent development exercise: Create a list of team members on your unit with potential for advancement or promotion. Don't forget to add your name to the list! Begin a conversation about succession planning with your nurse manager, and explore ways to help develop this talent within the unit, department, and organization. Identify and engage at least one person to coach, preceptor, or mentor. Perhaps the next executive nurse leader is even now one of your team members—perhaps it is you!—just waiting for the encouragement to take the next step in a career in leadership.

Problem Solving: Using Critical and Creative Thinking

Problems occur when there is a disconnect or difference between a current state and a goal state. *Problem solving* is the process used to close real or perceived gaps between present situations and desired goals, a situation not previously encountered, or a solution from past experiences. Once a gap is perceived, the problem-solving process is initiated, critical and creative thinking skills are accessed, and a solution is sought to fill the gap.

Critical thinking is a process for analyzing information to gain a deeper understanding of ideas and behaviors. It is purposeful, selective, orderly, predictable, planned, and analytical. It considers probabilities to help guide decisions and actions. You engage in critical thinking when you compare and contrast ideas, provide reasons for your thoughts, and evaluate situations and the ideas and actions of others. *Creative thinking* is seen when you generate new ideas, show originality, and flexibly shift your traditional perspectives. When you look outside the box to solve problems, apply your ideas in different contexts, develop your own stories, and think in unique ways, you are thinking creatively.

Hansel (1989) described seven steps to increase awareness of problems and how to articulate a way through them to resolution. It is a simple, clear approach to help you think critically and creatively problem solve:

1. Recognize and accept the problem (the most important step).

2. Analyze the problem; take it apart, simplify it, and carefully look at each part.

3. Define the problem; eliminate anything not needed, identify the issues, clarify the major goal(s). for solving the problem, and write out the problem or state it clearly.

4. Brainstorm as many ideas or potential solutions as possible.

5. Select the best possible way to solve the problem at this time.

6. Implement the selected best solution for the problem.

7. Evaluate the selected solution's effect or result. Did it correct the problem? If not, consider what could be done to improve the solution or select an alternative approach.

Much of a charge nurse leader's job is to identify and solve problems; it is a continuing process. Problems are simply challenges to be met and managed. They provide opportunities to identify innovative solutions for resolving conflict; for working with nurse managers to manage unit budgets, resources, and supplies; and, exploring ideas for working effectively with difficult employees, patients, or families.

Managing Conflict and Setting Boundaries

The better able team members are to engage, speak, listen, hear, interpret, and respond constructively, the more likely their teams are to leverage conflict rather than be leveled by it.

—*Runde and Flanagan*

Much like problems, conflict is inevitable though not always negative. In your role as charge nurse leader, you will encounter differences in opinions, ideas, methods, values, cultures, languages, perceived and real needs, ethics, and beliefs, which sometimes lead to incivility and intense disagreements. Negative conflict occurs when differences, concerns, and disagreements are ignored or poorly managed, resulting in increased stress, decreased productivity, loss of relevant information, disrupted decision-making processes and broken relationships, decreased patient safety and satisfaction, and wasted time and energy.

Sherman (2013) defines *civility* as the behaviors that show respect toward another person, make them feel valued, and contribute to mutual respect, effective communication, and team collaboration. *Workplace incivility* is low-intensity deviant behavior with ambiguous intent to harm another in violation of workplace norms for mutual respect; uncivil behaviors are characteristically rude and discourteous, displaying a lack of regard for others. *Positional violence* and *bullying* rise from negative conflict, often start with incivility, and may occur when staff members who were once peers refuse to respect or respond to you as a representative of the nurse manager for shift unit operations. Conflict must be handled quickly and positively before it reaches this level of aggression and negatively impacts staff engagement and patient safety.

When properly handled, conflict can have positive outcomes and and impact when it becomes the first step in facilitating innovative change and risk taking. It can pull team members together to work toward mutual goals and encourage interchanges of differing ideas, styles, methods, and approaches to providing patient-centered care. Positive conflict encourages teamwork and productivity, initiative, innovation, and risk taking to improve quality, safety, and practice outcomes.

Charge nurse leaders are often called to manage conflict and turn it into productive problem solving. You may not be able to resolve conflicts among team members or between staff and patients, but you may be able to help them work through their disagreements. Your responsibilities in managing conflict include the following:

- Identify real or potential conflict situations
- Establish boundaries
- Deal with conflict in its earliest stage
- Get issues, concerns, or needs out in the open
- Listen to but do not agree with each person's point of view
- Do not allow incivility or bullying
- Help people focus on constructive problem solving; redirect blaming or complaining
- Work with people to help them resolve their own conflicts, develop their own solutions, and take action to reduce or eliminate future conflict
- If the situation remains conflictual, engage the chain of command as appropriate (e.g., call the nurse manager or physician of record to address the remaining concerns or issues)

When we fail to set boundaries and hold people accountable, we feel used and mistreated. This is why we sometimes attack who they are, which is far more hurtful than addressing a behavior or a choice.

—Brené Brown

Boundaries are the spaces between authority and vulnerability, the formal and informal exercising of power. They define rules of who participates and how, setting the professional limits of relationships. Boundaries define healthy relationships for teams, leaders, patients, and others. They lower the risk to charge nurse leaders, staff and other team members, and patients by controlling power differentials, protecting vulnerable patients and staff, and protecting staff from becoming over-involved or uncivil. They also provide legal protection for patients and staff.

The most common boundary problem occurs when staff members challenge your authority for making decisions about schedules, staffing, and assignments, or providing constructive feedback for performance evaluations or appraisals. Blurred or non-existent boundaries impede your ability to effectively manage unit operations and staff performance when in the charge nurse leader role.

It is imperative that nurse managers and team members address the potential for incivility, bullying, and potential positional violence when conflict occurs before they become a real problem. These behaviors should never be tolerated or allowed to go unchecked. Strategies for promoting civility in the workplace and dealing with lateral and positional violence and bullying, limit setting and boundaries around the dual relationships you as a charge nurse leader maintain with your peers/staff should be folded into the charge nurse leader job description and functional statement. What does yours say?

The challenge in handling conflict and maintaining boundaries lies in trying to meet the personal and practical needs that are part of every interaction. The practical need is to resolve the conflict and the problems driving it. Generally, this is only possible if the following personal needs are first met:

- For each person to feel valued and respected
- To be heard and understood
- To contribute to the discussion and solution

As a charge nurse leader, you walk a tightrope when managing staff performance. This is possibly one of your most difficult and demanding roles. Charge nurse leaders facilitate, make important decisions, problem solve, manage conflict, and delegate assignments that affect the delivery of patient-centered care every shift. To do so effectively, professionally, and efficiently, you require support, resources, and continuous training. Talent development often begins with you, yielding a significant return on investment and expectations at the unit level as you move upward into ever more advanced leadership roles and positions.

Diversity of expertise and professional abilities are potential sources of conflict among team members. They may struggle over leadership, especially when status or power is confused with authority. Therefore, it is important to stay focused on patient-centered goals and to deal openly and constructively with the conflict through consistent communication and shared problem solving. Doing so contributes to your ability to work together to provide team-based care while building healthy teams. By attending to your staff members' practical and personal needs when managing conflict, setting boundaries, and shutting down incivility, bullying behaviors, and positional violence, you can facilitate more engaged, productive, and safe work teams.

4
Quality, Data, and Continual Improvement

It's the little things that make the big things possible. Only close attention to the fine details of any operation makes the operation first class.

—*J. Willard Marriott*

Role of Quality and Continual Improvement in Frontline Leadership

The organization defines quality but employees live it. To be successful in performance and process improvement, everyone must participate in quality management. As a charge nurse leader, you engage in activities and crucial actions needed to shift the organizational culture to excellence through relevant unit and work area operations.

You have already demonstrated your mastery of clinical skills, critical thinking, and collegial and collaborative team engagement. You have participated in professional development and provided patient-centered care in your units and practice areas. Although you may have collected data and responded to nursing-specific quality indicators, you may not have become involved in continuous process improvement (CPI) or quality improvement outside of your assigned work area. At this point, you need to know more about quality than can be found in the structure of the nursing care process (i.e., Subjective data collection, Objective data collection, Assessment, and Planning (SOAP) for patient care). The more common approach to quality and continual process improvement in healthcare is the Shewart model, or the Plan, Do, Check, Act (PDCA) model (see Figure 4.1). To clarify, let's begin with some definitions (Roth, 2015; Swihart & Figueroa, 2014).

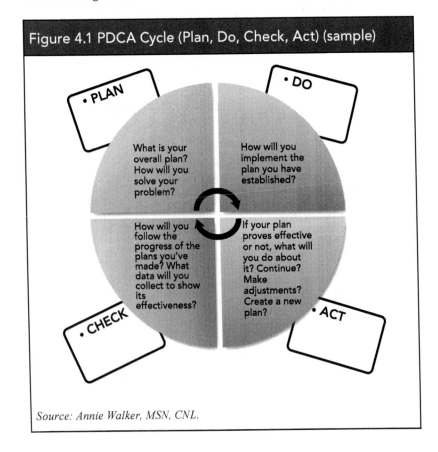

Figure 4.1 PDCA Cycle (Plan, Do, Check, Act) (sample)

• PLAN

What is your overall plan? How will you solve your problem?

• DO

How will you implement the plan you have established?

How will you follow the progress of the plans you've made? What data will you collect to show its effectiveness?

If your plan proves effective or not, what will you do about it? Continue? Make adjustments? Create a new plan?

• ACT

• CHECK

Source: Annie Walker, MSN, CNL.

Quality cannot be defined without context. It is determined by comparing a set of characteristics with a set of requirements and identifying the degree of compliance with that set of requirements (i.e., needs, expectations, or obligations). For example, charge nurse leaders and Clinical Nurse Leaders (CNL), build relationships and create interdisciplinary and interprofessional team activities in quality and continual improvement that do the right thing, at the right time, in the right way for the best possible outcomes (AHRQ, *www.ahrq.gov*).

The International Organization for Standardization (ISO, *www.iso.org*) describes the following eight basic principles of quality management, which are used to improve performance and process and to manage quality in all unit operations and coordination of patient-centered care:

1. *Customer focus*: Identify needs and requirements; exceed expectations through performance measures, assessments, and competency verifications; involve patients and families in team rounds and care meetings

2. *Leadership*: Establish unity of purpose and direction of unit operations and coordination of care delivery processes; maintain internal unit environment to achieve organization's objectives during the charge nurse leader training, orientation, and competency processes in partnership with managers, educators, staff and other team members, and human resources staff

3. *Involvement of people*: Have motivated, committed, engaged, empowered staff at all levels of organization (e.g., human resources, education, management and leadership, staff and other team members, faculty (for students), patients, and families)

4. *Process approach with process improvement*: When activities and related resources are managed as a process, a desired result is achieved more efficiently (e.g., expanding your training, orientation, and competency verifications as a frontline leader)

5. *System approach*: Identify, understand, and manage interrelated processes as a system; integrate quality preceptorships and shadowing experiences with CNLs into the mission, vision, and strategic planning processes for frontline leadership development and succession planning

6. *Continual improvement*: Set continual improvement as a permanent objective across the organization, and realize it within the microsystem of unit operations

7. *Factual approach to decision-making* based on analysis of data, evidence, and information (i.e., evidence-based practice, research, and practice-based evidence)

8. *Interdependent and mutually beneficial interdisciplinary and interprofessional relationships* to enhance your ability to create and sustain value, resource utilization, and cross-functional learning and competency activities (e.g., you may be called to assist on other units or to mentor other frontline leaders)

Quality management and continual improvement are critical considerations in the development of emerging nurse leaders such as you. You ensure interdisciplinary and interprofessional collaboration in all quality improvement (QI) activities. For example, you may facilitate or participate in the following:

- Monitoring nurse-sensitive quality indicators and reporting on performance measures

- Integrating safety priorities and relevant quality processes, functions, and services into continual improvement activities

- Engaging in peer review activities, data collection, and QI projects
- Attending quality councils and risk management committees
- Contributing to evidence-based design (EBD, e.g., noise, light, equipment, patient rooms, safe environments)
- Establishing and supporting unit-level journal clubs

You work with nurse managers, staff, and other team members to manage resources (human, financial, and materials) and risks for safe, efficient, quality outcomes. Your role in quality and continual improvement is pervasive and critical to the effectiveness and efficiency of unit operations and coordination of patient care. But you probably need a few tools to begin.

Using Tools for Continual Improvement

Review any standards, guidelines, or policies influencing quality, process, and safety on your unit. If you are fortunate enough to have a CNL, explore the available tools and processes that he or she uses for process and continual improvement within your unit. Include your nurse manager in the discussion, and consider tools already in place. For example, while there are many quality control tools available to improve performance, one of the most common ones used in healthcare is the Plan-Do-Check-Act (see Figure 4.1) model. This framework guides improvement by testing changes on a small scale. It is used to meet ISO (PDCA) standards, Lean-Six Sigma (LSS), and The Joint Commission requirements for quality and process improvement.

The following questions can help guide you when using the PDCA quality process and folding it into your work with nurse managers and supervisors, educators, team members and CNLs, and support staff to advance the development and improved outcomes of coordination and delivery of unit services:

- What are we trying to accomplish?
- How will we know that a change is an improvement?
- What changes can we make that will result in improvement?
- What outcomes are we trying to influence (e.g., nursing-sensitive quality indicators, risks, performance measures, medical errors, wandering patients, recent increase in falls, patient satisfaction)?

The PDCA allows the charge nurse leader program team to explore opportunities for improvement and to review program outcomes:

- Plan the process improvement; identify data to be collected (e.g., from strategic planning, root cause analyses, feedback, and performance evaluations)
- Do the improvement, data collection, and analysis
- Check the findings for process improvement based on change(s) implemented
- Act to hold the gain, sustain the outcome, and continue improvements as needed

Dashboards and scorecards are created as spreadsheets, charts, or graphs to disseminate large amounts of information in a more viewer-friendly format (see Figure 4.2). Composed of the many measures used to monitor a variety of factors that affect patient care and the unit's overall effectiveness, these tools streamline and disseminate current information about unit participation and progress related to unit- and facility-based quality improvement initiatives. Basic dashboards and scorecards are, therefore, a quick and easy way of staying informed on quality and performance improvement measures. Providing a real-time, visual display of feedback encourages better staff involvement in the performance and process initiatives that affect them, their patients, and their units. Now that you have the idea, how do you build a dashboard or scorecard? Check out *Instructions to Develop a Dashboard* at *www.cms.gov/Medicare/Provider-Enrollment-and-certification/QAPI/downloads/InstrDevDshbddebedits.pdf.*

Figure 4.2 Unit dashboard (sample)

Name	Short title explaining what you're measuring for improvement		Date 8/11/2015	SAIL/ PI?
Department	Your service line name goes here		Position	

Numerator	Denominator	Hi Lo, % #	Aim Goal	
Numerator is the smallest of the two numbers. E.g. Patients with wheelchairs instead of all patients	Denominator is the larger number. E.g. All patients	Hi Rate	Why do this project?	

Month	Num	Denom	Result	Base-Line	Thresh-old	Dept Goal	Notes
Oct	10	25	40.0%	70.0%	80.0%	90.0%	
Nov	12	22	54.5%	70.0%	80.0%	90.0%	
Dec	12	12	100.0%	70.0%	80.0%	90.0%	
Jan	17	24	70.8%	70.0%	80.0%	90.0%	
Feb	15	17	88.2%	70.0%	80.0%	90.0%	
Mar	18	19	94.7%	70.0%	80.0%	90.0%	
Apr				70.0%	80.0%	90.0%	
May				70.0%	80.0%	90.0%	
Jun				70.0%	80.0%	90.0%	
Aug				70.0%	80.0%	90.0%	
Sep				70.0%	80.0%	90.0%	

Figure 4.2 Unit dashboard (sample) (cont.)

Month	Num	Denom	Result	Base-Line	Thresh-old	Dept Goal	Notes
Q1	34	59	57.6%	70.0%	80.0%	90.0%	
Q2	50	60	83.3%	70.0%	80.0%	90.0%	
Q3	0	0	████	70.0%	80.0%	90.0%	
Q4	0	0	████	70.0%	80.0%	90.0%	
YTD	84	119	70.6%	70.0%	80.0%	90.0%	

Source: Annie Walker, MSN, CNL

When there is a problem, how do you and your team members prevent it from occurring again? How do you communicate or share it with others? In CPI, data is collected, analyzed, and applied to practice. Processes are applied to evaluate effectiveness and move patient-centered care and unit operations to excellence. You achieve all process improvement by establishing and managing expectations, effectiveness, evaluation, and excellence (Baird, 2011).

Collecting, Analyzing, and Applying Data to Practice

The most important practical lesson that can be given to nurses is to teach them what to observe.

—*Florence Nightingale*

Patient safety is woven into every aspect of unit operations and coordination and delivery of patient care. To support patient safety, charge nurse leaders must be transparent about unit performance measures, process improvements, data management, and reporting. Other key activities around patient safety include data collection, analysis, and applications of data to practice.

Charge Nurse Program Builder

Data collection is often assigned or delegated as part of an ongoing safety initiative for healthcare organizations. For example, The Joint Commission's National Patient Safety Goals (NPSG) compliance activities are often part of regular audits conducted on nursing units. Charge nurse leaders work with Clinical Nurse Leaders (CNL) to collect and analyze data for nursing quality indicators, performance measures, and other quality monitors to provide information to improve patient care and safety when applied to practice. Together you ensure that all unit patient care information is kept confidential, protected, and aligned with organizational policies and procedures. Although doing so can be more difficult with electronic medical records, you and your team members work closely with informatics and information technology specialists to ensure that computers and unit data are properly managed and protected.

Clinical Nurse Leaders, Partners in Quality Improvement

Quality within any healthcare system depends on improving patient outcomes, which rely on continual nursing professional development and overall improvements in system performance. One of your most important resources for managing such improvements is the CNL. This clinician is a Master's prepared Advanced Generalist nurse who builds quality measures in patient care outcomes and implements evidence-based practice principles at the clinical point of care and service. These outcomes align with the facility's goals and strategic plan and can positively impact patient care processes.

For example, when working in collaboration with a CNL, you can align the care team with strategic performance goals. CNLs and the Quality Systems team are important resources for strategic planning for quality and performance improvement (objectives, priorities, expectations, deliverables, and timelines). Working together, you can establish an infrastructure for engaging and motivating staff and other team members to work toward achieving improved patient care outcomes within the organization's measures of performance. Because you lead people and manage things, CPI only happens when everyone engages to improve management of operations and care delivery.

As the context of healthcare environments continually evolves and changes, your role becomes more complex and demanding. However, these growing challenges offer expanding opportunities for developing partnerships with your nurse manager, CNLs, and interprofessional team members to improve quality, practice, and competency in managing unit operations and coordinating patient care. By taking of advantage of these opportunities, you can help create a unit culture of safety, quality, and practice excellence.

5
Performance Evaluations

Trust gives you the permission to give people direction, get everyone aligned, and give them the energy to go get the job done. Trust enables you to execute with excellence and produce extraordinary results. As you execute with excellence and deliver on your commitments, trust becomes easier to inspire, creating a flywheel of performance.

—*Douglas Conant*

As a charge nurse leader, you work closely with nurse managers, educators, interprofessional partners, and team members to manage unit operations and healthcare teams and to coordinate the care delivered to patients safely, effectively, and efficiently. You perform skillful balancing acts every shift. You are responsible for patient outcomes; oversee delivery of care and documentation of unit operations and status of care; coordinate staffing, schedules, and assignments; oversee patient flow; orient and assess staff competencies; and manage unit conflict and stress among staff, caregivers, patients, and families.

Performance evaluations are another management function of monitoring and assessing planned activities to determine whether the employee has met established goals, objectives, and competencies (Osuagwu & Osuagwu, 2006). They serve as measures to assess competency, position-specific clinical and leadership knowledge and skills, and ability to promote a synergistic work environment for providing safe, quality, patient-centered care. Performance appraisals are tools intended to guide individuals motivated to perform at their highest levels and to develop their abilities in leadership, especially if they are interested in advancing their careers (Alvear, 2006).

Performance evaluations can seem nebulous at best and may be peer-based or folded into performance appraisals that assess how well you managed the unit in the nurse manager's absence or when combined with your own patient care assignments. You understand these nuances. But now you are asked to participate in performance evaluations for your staff. How does that work?

Team Roles in Performance Evaluations

Performance evaluations assess how duties are performed against a set standard of expectations and guided practice. Frequently, performance evaluations include input from team members and from peers, nurse managers, and staff. Other team members (e.g., educators, interdisciplinary team members, interprofessional partners, patients, and family members) may provide input as well.

Your leadership role comes with certain expectations of performance, delineated by the nurse manager. This is where a job description (see Figure 1.1) or functional statement can provide critical guidance. You serve as an authority working with the nurse manager, sometimes in their absence or when they are handling competing demands and higher-level facility obligations. You are assigned to manage nursing teams during your shifts by guiding, delegating, overseeing, and supporting unit or work area nursing staff and patient outcomes. You play a pivotal role in the success of the teams you lead.

Three primary groups participate in providing feedback and performance evaluation input for your performance evaluation:

1. Charge nurse leader: Peer (see Figure 5.1)

2. Nurse manager: Employee

3. Staff nurse: Subordinate team member

Figure 5.1 Charge nurse leader peer performance evaluation tool (sample)

Information
Charge nurse leader name: (Nurse manager to fill in name and distribute to random team members, both clinical and nonclinical)
Date of peer evaluation:
Name of evaluator:
NOTE: *All peer evaluation ratings and comments will be confidential and reviewed only by nurse manager.*
Rating scale and instructions
Using a scale of 1–3, assign the appropriate score in the rating box. If you score a 1 in any of the sections, please include a comment in the "Opportunities for Improvement" section.   1 = Inconsistently meets expectations   2 = Consistently meets expectations   3 = Exceeds expectations

Peer charge nurse leader performance element	Rating (1–3)	Opportunities for improvement
Approaches complex situations and changes with a positive attitude		
Inspires and supports team members' professional development		

Figure 5.1 Charge nurse leader peer performance evaluation tool (sample) (cont.)

Peer charge nurse leader performance element	Rating (1–3)	Opportunities for improvement
Is clinically knowledgeable and competent		
Is objective in all decision-making situations		
Is proactive and plans ahead		
Follows through on initiatives and keeps commitments		
Role models professional behavior		
Adheres to regulatory requirements, policies, procedures, and standards of practice		
Holds team members accountable for practice decisions and actions		
Shares clinical knowledge and expertise with other team members		
Actively listens to all participants during conflict		
Communicates clearly and accurately		
Manages time and resources effectively		
Manages stressful situations effectively		
Contributes to collaborative team-based care		
Engages in team building and collegiality		
Rounds with team members		
How would you most like to recognize this charge nurse leader peer? For what?		

Charge Nurse Program Builder

Figure 5.1 Charge nurse leader peer performance evaluation tool (sample) (cont.)
Additional comments

These team members demonstrate their level of cohesiveness, productivity, dynamics of unit working relationships, successful unit operations, and safe patient-centered care outcomes. Providing feedback and evaluating performance are critical in assessing your progress as charge nurse leader.

Types of Feedback and Performance Evaluations

The quality of our expectations determines the quality of our actions.

—Andre Godin, French socialist

Feedback and performance evaluations are closely related, but they are not the same. Performance evaluation begins with feedback that is specific, factual, descriptive, clearly understood, timed to be most useful, sensitive, constructive, and directed at behavior rather than at personality traits (Swihart & Figueroa, 2014). Feedback may be positive, negative, or constructive (see Figure 5.2). Performance evaluation is based on effective feedback. However, it is separate from the performance appraisal system, which determines whether an employee is meeting his or her contractual agreements with the organization. Feedback, verification, validation, results, and outcomes evaluation are terms often used to acknowledge the overlap of performance review and competency assessment (see Figure 5.3) and to clarify the important role of feedback.

Figure 5.2 Guidelines for providing effective feedback

Attributes of effective feedback:

*Specific, not general	*Descriptive, not judgmental	*Timed to be most useful	*Constructive, not destructive
*Factual, not opinionated	*Clearly understood by the receiver	*Sensitive to preceptee's feelings and needs	*Directed at behavior, not at personalities
*Share information, not give advice	*Based on mutual rapport and trust	*Allows for preceptee's perspective	*Leads to positive outcomes

Elements of feedback:

Describe what was observed: who, what, when, where, and how.	Description: "After loosening the dressing, you put on sterile gloves and removed the old dressing."
Relate how the observed behavior made you feel.	Reaction: "I felt that the sterile field had been violated. This is the reason I suggested that you discard the clean dressing."
Be as specific as possible, Avoid judging and generalizing.	Specifics: "The gloves you used to pick up the new sterile dressing were the same as those you used to discard the old soiled dressing. A non-sterile surface came into contact with a sterile surface."
Suggest an alternative action, behavior, or response.	Alternative behavior: "Another way to manage this situation is to remove the gloves when you discard the soiled dressing and wash your hands. Then put on another pair of gloves before handling the instruments and sterile surface."

Principles of providing feedback:

Positive: Whenever possible, provide positive feedback.
Constructive: When necessary, provide constructive feedback.

Figure 5.2 Guidelines for providing effective feedback (cont.)

Negative: Unless an emergency situation arises, avoid giving negative feedback.

B.E.E.R. feedback model:

B: Behavior	What is the preceptee doing or not doing that is unacceptable?
E: Effect	Why is the behavior unacceptable? How does it hurt productivity, impact safe patient care, breach policies and procedures, bother others, and so on?
E: Expectation	What does the preceptor expect the preceptee to do or not do to change?
R: Result	What will happen if the preceptee changes (positive tone) or this behavior continues (negative tone)?

Figure 5.3 Performance rating scale (sample)

Performance rating scale

Excellent performance	Good performance	Average performance	Poor performance
The charge nurse leader:	The charge nurse leader:	The charge nurse leader:	The charge nurse leader:
❑ Consistently functions with minimal need for guidance, except in unusual work situations.	❑ Generally functions with minimal need for guidance in most work situations.	❑ Generally functions with a moderate amount of guidance in most work situations.	❑ Functions only with direct supervision in most work situations.
❑ Consistently performs work tasks safely.	❑ Usually performs tasks safely.	❑ Usually performs tasks safely.	❑ Tasks not performed safely or done with difficulty.
❑ Consistently integrates position-specific knowledge with skills.	❑ Usually integrates position-specific knowledge with skills.	❑ Requires some assistance in integrating position-specific knowledge with skills.	❑ Requires frequent assistance to integrate position-specific knowledge with skills.
❑ Initiates requests for new learning opportunities.	❑ Recognizes need to learn new skills but needs encouragement.	❑ Recognizes need to learn new skills but needs specific direction.	❑ Unable to recognize the need to learn new skills or knowledge.
❑ Applies position-specific knowledge appropriate to assigned unit or work area.	❑ Generally applies position-specific knowledge appropriate to assigned unit or work area.	❑ Demonstrates an average level of knowledge appropriate to the unit or work area.	❑ Requires detailed instructions to use position-specific knowledge appropriate to unit or work area.

When participating in performance evaluations, consider the following questions about yourself and your staff:

1. If there is a position description for the role, are you and your staff doing what you were selected to do?

2. Do you function below, at, or above set expectations?

3. Do you competently and safely function in your clinical and leadership roles?

4. What are you doing particularly well?

5. What do you need to change?

6. What might you do differently to improve in your assigned duties?

7. What training and development do you need to perform your assigned duties?

8. What other questions might help you assess performance?

Feedback is provided more frequent than performance evaluations; and is intended to reflect, document, and modify performance. You should provide ongoing feedback and discuss improvements and progress based on that feedback. Improved performance is a critical addition to performance evaluations.

When conveyed with supportive language, feedback encourages you and your staff members to experience successes, maintain motivation, reinforce desired performance, and correct unsatisfactory behaviors. Provide frequent feedback and discuss whether the feedback was positive, negative, or constructive. What were the attributes and elements of the feedback? Consider the BEER (Behavior, Effect, Expectation, and Result) feedback model from business and how feedback is reflected in the performance evaluation process (see Figure 5.2) (Swihart & Gantt, 2015).

Performance Evaluation Process

Performance evaluations usually include written objectives, a timeline with specification of learning activities and competencies to be assessed when, where, and by whom, and what tools will be used. There are essentially four steps in the performance evaluation process (Swihart & Figueroa, 2014; Swihart & Gantt, 2015):

1. Measurement of a behavioral competency, action, skill, or ability

2. Comparison of the expected action or behavior against an established standard of performance for that competency

3. Verification of effect; did the observed response meet the standard of performance?

4. A decision is based on the assessment and verification processes and the result or outcome documented

Stated understanding or learning cannot be directly observed. Performance evaluation requires observable and measurable behaviors, skills, actions, or abilities. Improved performance is inferred based on changed behavior, increased competency, and application to practice. Without a basis for comparison of the desired competency, it cannot be measured objectively. Written objectives and criteria make the standard for satisfactory performance evident for you, your staff, the nurse manager, and other stakeholders.

Consider some of the following tips for successful performance evaluations and, ultimately, excellent performance appraisals.

Taking Charge: Tips for Successful Charge Nurse Leaders

Being a charge nurse leader is a challenging task for many; moreover, being a *successful* charge nurse leader warrants an elevated level of commitment and a skillful sustained effort. The following tips and accountability strategies may help (Swihart & Gantt, 2015):

1. Keep portfolios, logs, or journals of progress with notes on accomplishments; reflective discussions; responses to feedback from peers, managers, and team members; personal and professional goals and objectives; career plans; guidance from coaches, preceptors, and mentors; and opportunities to grow and develop further.

2. Assist nurse managers with unit operations and coordination of care; extend their leadership, authority, and efficiency as frontline leaders. Use your clinical expertise and knowledge to advocate for staff and other team members in negotiating resources, collaborating across service lines, and managing unit and patient situations as they arise.

3. Be optimistic and visionary, maintaining a positive attitude.

4. Work hard and set good examples. Attend to details while exploring the larger picture.

5. Network within the organization and department; volunteer to work on unit and central shared governance councils, safety committees, and problem-solving task teams; and establish a peer network. Strategic positioning may help with proactive and preemptive solutions to increase unit productivity, improve quality and processes, lower unit costs, and increase staff and patient satisfaction.

6. Be professionally active in local and national professional organizations, attend workshops and seminars, write articles,

participate in a unit journal club, and monitor trends and issues in nursing and leadership.

7. Role model professionalism through self-respect, excellence in clinical and leadership decisions and actions, and demonstrated professional integrity. Treat everyone with courtesy, consideration, compassion, and respect.

8. Provide realistic feedback and encouragement. Acknowledge subordinates and team members for good performance. Describe the action or behavior, and reinforce the positive. Celebrate successes whenever possible and appropriate.

9. Think carefully and rationally before writing or speaking. Hasty words and deeds can do more harm than good, and unintended consequences can create an uncomfortable and even hostile work setting. Set boundaries and hold to them, especially when managing conflict or stressful situations. When mistakes occur, acknowledge them, take ownership of them, and correct them. Relationships are far more important than egos.

10. Keep an open mind when communicating with others. Allow the free flow of information with candor, respect, and equity, but within limits. For example, set boundaries for disclosures, and limit personal sharing. Avoid critical language, negatives, and absolutes in conversations. The nursing unit is one of safety and not of blame; maintain that safety in all communications and behaviors. Be tactful, honest, and direct. Deliver every message with compassion and genuineness.

11. When faced with unsettling or difficult ethical dilemmas, explore ways to resolve them.

12. Demonstrate genuine interest and concern for staff and team members; ask them how their work is going, and actively listen to their responses. Be receptive to and supportive of

ideas and suggestions for improved services or operations. Share relevant information, and seek their input. Give immediate feedback regarding how their input anticipated or solved a unit or patient problem.

13. NEVER tolerate incivility, bullying, hostility, or violence in the workplace. This includes inflammatory or derogatory verbal or nonverbal language.

14. Maintain a good sense of humor to stay centered, balanced, and relaxed.

15. Use a participatory management style for unit operations and coordination of care delivery. Ensure staff have been coached or trained to participate and to contribute meaningfully. Share ownership, responsibility, accountability, and outcomes with staff and team members equitably.

16. Use staff meetings to encourage staff input in developing unit objectives, identifying competencies, problem solving, and decision-making for improving unit productivity, eliminating waste, and reducing costs. Give prompt feedback for any ideas or suggestions they provide and related outcomes. Include the nurse manager and other team members when appropriate.

As a frontline leader, you require a degree of authority, critical thinking skills, credibility, accurate clinical judgment, and effective communication to ensure that the highest level of safe, quality care is provided to patients within your units and practice settings. Further strategies for success include charge nurse leader training combining didactic content with a preceptorship to help you build leadership competency prior to taking on this critical role. Moreover, nurse leaders are needed to help develop strategic guidelines, position statements and descriptions, and competencies. These would expand skill sets and leadership activities to produce more competent, empowered, and resourceful frontline leaders.

6

Charge Nurse Leaders Caring for Self and Others

When we long for life without difficulties, remind us that oaks grow strong in contrary winds and diamonds are made under pressure.

—Peter Marshall, Scottish clergyman, 1902–1949

Managing Stress

The interpretation of stressful events is more important than the events themselves.

—Richard Lazarus

Before you can manage stress, you must first understand what it is and what it is not. Lazarus (1986), a behavioral and cognitive psychologist, seems to capture the essence of stress when he calls it a condition or feeling experienced when one perceives demands exceed the resources the person can access or mobilize, when he or she feels out of control. Sound familiar? The effects of stressful encounters build quickly. People respond differently in how they handle stress in different situations, reporting numerous emotional and physical disorders linked to it (American Institute of Stress, *www.stress.org/stress-effects/*). Everyone reacts to personal and work stressors—even those who generally handle stress more effectively feel more comfortable in their positions and lived experiences, express more confidence in their knowledge and skills, and believe they can meet any event competently.

There are two common models used to describe the instinctive reactions people have to short-term or long-term stress:

- Short-term stress: Walter Cannon's (1930) theory of *acute stress response*, or *fight or flight*, a response that enables someone to use a lot of energy rapidly to cope with perceived or real threats to survival or sudden shocks. This can cause irritability and overreaction (e.g., during conflicts with others or last-minute deadlines or sudden changes in patient status).

- *Long-term stress*: Hans Selye's (1907–1982) developed the General Adaptation Syndrome (GAS), a stress model that describes three predictable stages for how the body responds to long-term exposure to stress:

  1. Alarm stage: Body has a burst of energy and reacts to the stressor

  2. Resistance stage: Body attempts to resist or adapt to stressor(s), gradually depleting physical and emotional resources

  3. Exhaustion stage: Energy is depleted, and normal functioning no longer possible; fight-or-flight responses over time can lead to this stage of GAS

How you manage varying levels and degrees of stress and stressors is part of frontline leadership. You assess situations and events to determine whether they are threatening in any way, such as a time interruption when patient care rounding has begun or an angry complaint from the nurse manager triggers the fight-or-flight response). If the interruption is a report on one of the patients, you may deem it important and manage the stress more effectively. However, it may be more difficult to manage the stress if the nurse manager's angry complaints focus on how you handled the interruption. Stressors differ for everyone.

It is important to identify activities that promote relaxation, stress reduction, and rebalancing and to engage in them amidst the many competing demands on your time and energy each day. Healing and renewing activities may be grounded in participating in recreational events, attending theater and engaging in the arts, expressing your faith, or simply slipping away from the daily grind and reconnecting with the divine. Your ability to manage stress extends to recognizing and supporting your strengths and finding assistance in meeting challenges at each opportunity, as in the following examples:

1. Engage in peer discussions and debriefings for solving problems and celebrating successes

2. Clearly delineate and separate your role, work expectations, responsibilities, accountabilities, and competencies

3. Do not be afraid or hesitant to ask for help

4. Communicate, communicate, communicate

5. Be respectful and professional

6. Forgive and let go when appropriate

7. Leave work at work—delegate!

8. Accept what cannot be changed

9. Create lists for "MUST do" and "MIGHT do (if there is time)" and "will NEVER do!"

10. Revise expectations regularly and as needed

11. Relax and renew energies and creativity

12. Nurture a deep seated and refreshing sense of humor

13. Organize and make time for your personal priorities (e.g., family, friends, work, school, faith)

Stress impacts your ability to learn, to interact with others reasonably and kindly, and to do your job effectively. It can damage health, relationships, and futures—or it can drive you to succeed. You must discover how to manage stress and redirect it into positive and challenging opportunities to change outcomes. Stress is generated by how circumstances are approached and interpreted. David Allen observed, "Much of the stress that people feel doesn't come from having too much to do. It comes from not finishing what they've started." Stress can be a powerful driving force in many ways (e.g., to improve skills and abilities and move into ever-greater leadership responsibilities). It all depends on how you approach it and how resilient you can be.

Developing Resiliency

Resiliency is the capacity to recover quickly from difficulties, the ability to toughen and spring back. The brain can be rewired to become more resilient to the negative effects of stress (Goewey, 2014). There are methods of extinguishing stress reactions and amplifying higher brain function linked to success in life, joy at work, and peace at home. One method is through self-regulation. Take time to reset and recalculate. From the day-to-day stressors encountered, you can become immunocompromised and more prone to sickness, illness, and disease. The heart-brain connection leads to cognitive inhibition and may cause you to say or do things you would not ordinarily say or do.

Therefore, it is imperative you self-regulate, regenerate, and recharge your batteries. You need to be able to focus energy to achieve balance between heart, mind and emotions, and spirit, aligning them and making sure they are in sync through focused breathing and spending time in positive environments with positive thoughts and positive people to build up energy reserves and resiliency. Research has demonstrated that forgiveness, releasing bitterness and anger, and dealing positively and proactively with stressors can build resiliency and balance within (Lackey, 2014) by learning to care for yourself psychologically, physically, and spiritually.

Caring for Self Psychologically, Physically, and Spiritually

Healing ourselves is pivotal to healing others.
—*Kim Richards*

The American Nurses Association (ANA, n.d.) describes healthy nurses as those who actively focus on creating and maintaining a balance and synergy of physical, intellectual, emotional, spiritual, personal, and professional well-being. They live life to the fullest across the wellness/illness continuum as they become stronger role models, advocates, and educators, for themselves, their families, their communities and work environments, and ultimately for their patients. This description implies nurses must take an active role in maintaining their own health—the physical, emotional, and spiritual demands of the profession are great and will affect their health adversely without proactive measures (Letvak, 2014).

Your role as the charge nurse leader is complex, with unit responsibilities that include oversight of patient care, managing staff interactions, and documentation and reporting of daily unit activities. You are in a key position to influence and promote change. At the same time, you are expected to lead staff while managing the work systems and processes on your unit to ensure that patient and staff needs are met. No wonder you are stressed!

Eleanor Brownn reminds us that "You cannot serve from an empty vessel." To be genuinely effective, you must take time for intentional self care to renew your energies and avoid burnout and ill health. Sherman (2013) shared five more reasons why investing in self care is important:

1. *Rest is an investment in yourself, your team, and your future.* Rest is critical for physical, emotional, and spiritual health. It allows you to be more alert and better able to process the many personal and professional challenges you confront.

2. *Recharging your battery will make you a better leader.* Time taken to recharge and renew energy makes you a stronger and better leader and reduces the likelihood of burnout.

3. *Find an activity outside of work that brings self-renewal.* You need time to consistently and frequently engage in at least one activity outside of work that quiets the mind, soothes the spirit, and re-energizes, such as meditation, exercise, walking, reading, art, cooking, or prayer.

4. *Make time to reflect on how you use your time and energy at work.* Time in self-reflection is an important step in rebalancing work and life.

5. *Charge nurse leaders set the example for self care on their teams.* To achieve a healthy work environment, you need to promote the idea of self care. Role modeling is a powerful way to do this. Paying attention to your own self care will help keep you and your team members vibrant, and it will establish self care as a strong value in your work culture.

Self care creates balance, enhances well-being, reduces fatigue and burnout, and allows you to role model healthy behaviors by maintaining a balance between the demands of work and personal renewal activities. You create a culture of caring and rediscovery related to shared values, goals, creativity, and productivity. You will be less vulnerable to exhaustion, stress, and burnout as your expressions of intentional self care become a natural part of your life at home and at work.

Intentional self care

Personal health and self-renewal are priorities you pass on to your team members. Self-renewal fosters a state of well-being and includes health-promoting activities as determined by the individual. It requires accepting responsibility for one's own feelings and engaging the physical, psychological, mental, social, and spiritual dimensions of being. Eliminating negative self-talk and choosing to feel good about one's self and others are intentional decisions to help move one beyond adversities or competing demands that interfere with caring for self. Such activities are critical for increasing well-being and reducing and controlling stress (Antai-Otong, 2001).

Before you can adequately care for and guide others, you need to take care of yourself. Intentional self care provides opportunities to reduce negative stress and restore and maintain a state of holistic well-being. For example, relaxation techniques might include deep abdominal breathing, progressive relaxation, visualization and imagery, meditation, and grounding techniques. Antai-Otong (2001) and Mashburn (2015) describe many more activities to help you find renewal, refresh your energy, and reclaim your enthusiasm:

- Establish a regular exercise program
- Eat a balanced diet
- Take lunch breaks away from the work station or area

- Establish a regular sleeping pattern
- Comply with medical regimens, including diet and medications
- Visit dentists and healthcare providers regularly
- Take at least a week-long vacation or holiday annually
- Relax with music
- Decompress—take advantage of alone time
- Integrate quiet time at the beginning of the day
- Allow a time for space at the end of the work day
- Spend a few minutes performing mindless activities
- Work in a garden
- Rehydrate—drink plenty of water
- Get a massage or pedicure—or both!
- Spend time in the outdoors
- Pray and meditate
- Visualize a soothing place (beach, mountain stream, field covered in flowers)
- Do relaxation exercises whenever and wherever you can

Intentional self care is a gift. It is an unselfish act and practice of great benefit. Self-care activities at work include a conscious awareness of using time wisely, knowing when to delegate, knowing when to say no, setting limits, and laughing profoundly. No one can provide self care to anyone else. It can only be done and achieved by self. It requires making the decision and being committed to a lifestyle change to function at your best with the ability to always give your best.

Understanding how you are designed with the complexities of your unique qualities and integrated possibilities folded into a physical, social, psychological, and spiritual package helps you consider the best way to incorporate caring into the renewal process. As a charge nurse leader, you must recognize and communicate your own needs to their leaders, peers, and team members. Stress management is a fundamental part of leadership and service. You need to develop and implement a plan to ensure self-renewal and support in the workplace while you are engaged in frontline leadership, unit operations, and coordination of care delivery while managing stressful situations and events.

This chapter is only a brief exploration of what self care means and offers a few ideas for engaging in intentional self care. It is only meant to open a few doors and encourage you to find what you need to fill your vessel to overflowing. As the benefits of self-renewal are realized, a culture of caring for self and others can expand connections with colleagues, staff and other team members, patients, and families. Through you, your unit can become a place of renewal and comradery, a psychologically and spiritually safe place to work and grow.

Bibliography

1. Alvear, J. (2006). *Manager's guide to performance appraisals. FastFacts, 2,* 1–2. Retrieved from http://www.chcf.org/~/media/MEDIA%20LIBRARY%20Files/PDF/F/PDF%20FFGuidePerformanceAppraisals.pdf.

2. American Nurses Association. (June 29, 2012). *The Supreme Court Decision matters for Registered Nurses, their families and patients.* Retrieved from http://www.emergingrnleader.com/wp-content/uploads/2012/07/SupremeCourtDecision-Analysis.pdf.

3. American Nurses Association. (ANA, 2012). *Principles for nurse staffing (2nd ed.).* American Nurses Association: Silver Spring, MD.

4. American Nurses Association. (ANA, 2015). *The code of ethics with interpretative statements.* American Nurses Association: Silver Spring, MD.

5. American Nurses Association (n.d.). *HealthyNurse.* Retrieved from www.nursingworld.org/MainMenuCategories/WorkplaceSafety/Healthy-Nurse.

6. Antai-Otong, D. (October 2001). Critical incident stress

debriefing: A health promotion model for workplace violence. *Perspectives in Psychiatric Care, 37*(4), 125–132.

7. Baird, K. (2011). *Raising the bar on service excellence: The health care leader's guide to putting passion into practice.* eBookIt.com: Amazon Digital Services, Inc.

8. Black, J. S. & Gregersen, H. B. (2008). *It starts with one: Changing individuals changes organizations (2nd ed.).* Upper Saddle River, JN: Pearson Education, Inc.

9. Gantt, K. (2014). Ethics in preceptoring. In *The Preceptor Program Builder: Essential Tools for a Successful Preceptor Program* by D. Swihart and S. Figueroa. Danvers, MA: HCPro.

10. Goewey, D. J. (2014). *The end of stress.* Beyond Word Publishing/Atria Books: Hillsboro, OR.

11. Hansel, T. (1989). *Eating problems for breakfast: A simple, creative approach to solving any problem (a classic).* Nashville, TN: W. Publishing Group.

12. Institute for Healthcare Improvement. (IHI, 2003). Optimizing patient flow: moving patients smoothly through acute care settings. *IHI Innovation Series* white paper. Boston: Institute for Healthcare Improvement. Retrieved from http://www.ihi. org/resources/Pages/IHIWhitePapers/Optimizing Patient FlowMovingPatientsSmoothlyThrough AcuteCareSettings. aspx.

13. Lackey, D. (2014). *Self-regulation and heart rate variability coherence: Promoting psychological resilience in healthcare leaders.* Lisle, IL: Benedictine University.

14. Lazarus, R. S. (1986). *Psychological stress and the coping process (a classic).* New York, NY: McGraw-Hill.

15. Letvak, S. (September 30, 2014). Overview and Summary: Healthy Nurses: Perspectives on Caring for Ourselves. *The Online Journal of Issues in Nursing, 19*(3). Retrieved from

http://www.nursingworld.org/MainMenuCategories/ ANAMarketplace/ANAPeriodicals/OJIN/TableofContents/Vol-19-2014/No3-Sept-2014/OS-Healthy-Nurses.html.

16. Makaroff, K.S., Storch, J., Pauly, B., Newton, L. (2014). Searching for ethical leadership in nursing. *Nursing Ethics, 21*(6), 642–648.

17. Mashburn, J. (2015). Preceptor self-care and renewal. In J. W. Roth's *Core curriculum for preceptor advancement.* Sponsored by the American Academy for Preceptor Advancement. eBookIt.com: Amazon Digital Services, Inc.

18. Osuagwu, C. C., & Osuagwu, G. (2006). *From staff nurse to manager: A guide to successful role transition.* Booksurge. Available at www.booksurge.com.

19. Porter-O'Grady, T. (2003). A different age for leadership, part 1. *Journal of Nursing Administration, 33*(10), 105-110.

20. Roth, J. W. (Sr. Ed.). (2015). *Core curriculum for preceptor advancement.* Sponsored by the American Academy for Preceptor Advancement. eBookIt.com: Amazon Digital Services, Inc.

21. Sherman, R. O. (July 2012). 5 ways the Affordable Care Act could change nursing. *The Emerging RN Leader.* Retrieved from http://www.emergingrnleader.com.

22. Sherman, R. O. (2013). *2011-2013: The best of emerging RN leader blogs.* Retrieved from http://www.emergingrnleader. com/.

23. Sherman, R. O., Schwarzkopf, R., & Kiger, A. J. (February 2013). What we learned from our charge nurses. *Nurse Leader,* 34–39.

24. Swihart, D., & Figueroa, S. (2014). *The preceptor program builder: Essential tools for a successful preceptor program.* Danvers, MA: HCPro.

25. Swihart, D., & Gantt, K. (2015). *The charge nurse leader program builder: A competency-based approach.* Danvers, MA: HCPro.

26. Tanzi, D. (2015). Chapter 9. Communication. In the Core Curriculum for Preceptor Advancement by J. W. Roth, Sr. Editor. Sponsored by the American Academy for Preceptor Advancement. eBookIt.com: Amazon Digital Services, Inc.

27. U.S. Department of Health & Human Resources. (AHRQ, n.d.). PCMH. Agency for Healthcare Research and Quality. Retrieved from https://pcmh.ahrq.gov/.

28. Wright, D. (2002). *R + A + A: The secret formula for making communication and delegation easier.* Video 4 in the Moments of Excellence video series. Minneapolis: Creative Health Care Management.